Anxiety and Depression from a Patient's Perspective

ISBN: 10-1452884137
ISBN-13: 9781452884134

Anxiety and Depression from a Patient's Perspective

Richard Wyrabkiewicz

This book will definitely help people with anxiety and depression, Most of this is not from a professional or doctor's point of view or his or her conclusions. This book will give you the tools to help your negative thoughts and how to overcome anxiety in most cases; it will describe what depression is and how it will affect you. It is from my very own experience and conclusions. This book is very short and to the point and will definitely help you.

Dedication

This is dedicated to all the people living with anxiety and depression.

I am hoping this book will help you and that other people will have a better understanding of what you are going through.

What causes anxiety and depression and some methods to overcome and help?

Knowing there are millions of people with the same problem.

To my wife who endured with me when I have gone through some tough times.

Also to my daughter Kathaleen, I hope that she will understand her dad better and that she will always be "daddy's little girl.

Acknowledgement

Special thanks to **Mary Wallace** who read drafts on this book and gave me some good advice.

Dr. Kalib Kafaji clinical psychologist who inspired me to write this book and taught me how to eradicate negative thoughts with positive affirmations,.

Jeff Frost for his patience and all the time he spent with me using his computer knowledge. I could not have completed this Book without his help and skills.

Liz Potter Special thanks to Liz for sentence structure.

Table of Contents

I am Richard Wyrabiewicz and I was born on July 3,1951, I am writing to let you know that I have been suffering from anxiety for many years and later in life I would have depression episodes. I can remember developing some negative thought patterns as a little child. Abnormal thoughts and fears would enter my mind, unlike many children, I was unable to shake them off. I never talked with people about the thoughts and anxieties I was having.

At this young age I had already developed" flight or fright" patterns and I did not know what was going on..

CHAPTER 1

When I Was Young

I t all started when I was about ten and in the fifth grade. I recall it went something like this. My friend and I used to ride around the schoolyard on our bikes. We did this pretty often in the summer when school was out. There happened to be an apple tree in the yard of one of the nearby houses. This particular tree had branches that reached over the fence of the owner's yard and into the school grounds. So naturally, we would stand up on our bikes and try to pick the apples, which is common for boys to do. We did this a few times without a problem. But one day, it was almost as if the man who lived there was waiting for us.

There I was, in an awkward position on my bike. I had completely stopped to stand up and pick the apples. All of a sudden, my friend saw him and took off on the bike just before me As he was yelling something to me. My back was facing the man as he was running toward me. The man was right behind me yelling at me. I remember that distinctly to this day. My heart started beating faster and faster! I was trying to peddle faster and faster, but I was barely moving because I was so scared. I felt I was going as fast as I could. I remember his face and how mean he looked. He grabbed my bike. I was really scared. He held on to my ear saying, "I'm going to pull your ear off." The face he was making scared me half to death. His eyes were so big and round. They were just staring at me. I can't remember what else he said, but finally he let me go.

When I got home, I didn't say anything to my parents; maybe that's where I made my mistake. I felt that they would not have known what to say to me. Instead of this just being a normal situation that a kid would get into and forget about. My mind obsessed over it. I kept seeing his face over and over. I kept thinking about him pulling on my ear and yelling at me. For many days, that incident was the only thing on my mind. I didn't know what was going on. I thought it was normal to obsess over that type of incident. The obsessive thoughts were already in my life. There I was, ten years old, and the fears and anxieties were already at work. Unlike most kids, I didn't laugh this off. Clearly to this day, Thirty-eight years later, as I write this, I still remember the man's face as he was coming after me. Was this a normal reaction for a scared ten year old?

I remember a day when two teenagers got into a fight on the school grounds after school. One of them was bleeding badly from one eye. I knew this boy. He was kind of a friend. He never bothered me but he could be a bully to some. His eye was almost closed. The guy that hit him was a punk. He was there waiting for my friend when the last bell rang. Just as my friend came out, the other kid approached him. My friend was not the type to back down, so they fought! As the fight went on, my sixth grade teacher came out and clinched each one of the boys by the neck, and quickly stormed into the office with them.

My mind was filled with fear and anxiety. It was almost as though I was in the fight. I knew I was different from most boys, because even at that young of an age, fighting bothered me. I thought people should not hurt each other. What was I afraid of? I didn't know this pattern would follow me all my life. I guess I was born with an unnatural sensitivity that a lot of boys are not born with.

I remember another incident when I was in the sixth grade, as I was coming home from school. A boy I knew was beating up another friend of mine who didn't want to fight. The boy kept egging him on, knowing that eventually he would get mad enough and fights back.

He knew he could take my friend easily and wanted him to fight back. Finally, he had enough of the name calling and teasing: he fought back, and got badly beaten. He was crying. I felt so sorry for him. Other boys were making fun of him. I had that same fear I had before. I did not know that fear caused anxiety or does anxiety cause fear?

Other than the fears I was a normal kid with friends who enjoyed playing with other kids. Another friend and I were the two fastest runners in school. God blessed me with a good pair of legs. That was one thing I was very proud of. I didn't have girlfriends like some of my friends. I was shy and quiet. My thoughts were on other things. As I can recall, I never stole anything out of a store, not even a piece of candy, nor did I steal from anybody or try to hurt them in any way. I remember this boy coming into our class in the sixth grade who was from the Dominican Republic..I remember that some of the boys I hung around with started steering him the wrong way. He was a nice kid and I tried to keep him out of mischief. He was picking up some bad traits so I tried to talk to him, but he wouldn't listen. I often wonder about him and how his life turned out.

As I entered the seventh grade, I knew I was different. I had a very hard time getting used to all the different classes and I was missing my old friends. Everyone made new friends and kept their old ones. Everyone went into different classes every hour. I didn't like the change either. I felt an emptiness I had never felt before. This was the first time in my life I was forced to make a change. I have a hard time with change, and to this day, at Fifty-eight years old, I still have a hard time with change. To tell you more about my personality, here are some examples of how I don't like change:

I have had the same job for forty years.
I have been married to my wife for thirty-six years.
I have lived in the same house for thirty years.
I keep the same vehicle for five to eight years.

So I was, in the seventh grade. It seemed like I completely lost all confidence in myself what little confidence I had to begin with. I was in a new school with new classes, teachers, subjects, and students. At first, going through the changing of schools, I felt like I was lost. It was a new way of life. This is really when my thoughts and emotions started changing drastically. I found myself confused in class. There were other things running through my mind. I couldn't focus or concentrate very long without thinking about other things. Up to this point, there were no physical symptoms in my life, just anxious thoughts. Of course, at this point, I had no knowledge of what was triggering these thoughts. I had not read any material on anxiety, nor was I getting any psychotherapy to rectify the thoughts. I never knew there was treatment for this problem. The medicine now is so much more advanced that it was in the sixties. In those days when you went to a psychiatrist people thought you were different. It wasn't like it is today where ten percent or more of the people in the U.S. visit a psychiatrist once or more in their lives. In fact, it is gaining more and more acceptance every day.

CHAPTER 2

Brain Waves

I now have learned from reading that much of my problem was, and is to this day, a problem with brain-wave cycles. Let me explain what I mean. The average person, at an average time, during an average day, is at the Beta area, producing 21 cycles per second or CPS. When excited by anger, fear, nervousness or any stirring emotion, that rhythm increases and the brain activity rises to 22, 25 or more CPS. Poor health, excitability, poor learning ability and weak concentration are due in part to an excessive degree of brain-wave activity. The rhythm of good health, the rhythm of intelligence, the rhythm of concentration, the rhythm of pure genius is in the area of the brain wave production that falls below 19 cycles per second. Stress and anxiety are associated with a brain wave production of about 21 CPS. When brain wave activity is above 21 CPS, concentration is ruined. The thoughts of the individual go through an upheaval and are barraged by a series of inconsequential matters. Thousands of constantly changing thoughts, seemingly out of control, keep the mind from concentrating on what is important. In the high Beta area, 40 CPS, it becomes increasingly difficult to concentrate on any one subject for long. The mind flits from thought to thought like a bee buzzing from flower to flower. Before the complete formation of one thought, you're on to still another. It's difficult to remember things in the high beta area. This information was taken from the book: *You Can't Afford the Luxury Of A Negative Thought* by Peter McWilliams.

This was my problem all the way through school, and still is today. My brain waves are in the high Beta area. My mind goes from one thought to another. This explains my life and why I still have so much difficulty studying. Sometimes my mind is like a bee buzzing from flower to flower. Did I develop this problem early in youth or was I born with it? I'm still not sure.

I remember as a young boy, sitting on the couch putting together a model car. I liked doing that. I remember clearly after a few days of working on the car that it became really boring. So unintentionally, I started making things up in my mind. I actually created things and then started thinking about them. You know how creative kids can be! The thought patterns got worse as I got older. If I had known what the problem was, it may not have morphed into the situation it did.

Now imagine yourself having this problem in junior high school. For three years, you try to study hard, and still fail the tests. You read the material over and over and still have a hard time comprehending. You try to take notes as your teacher is lecturing and your mind goes from thought to thought. It became very frustrating for me. I tried hard to get good grades, but I really did not know how to study for the tests. Later, in high school, I learned how to study and also realized I had to memorize a lot of the material in order to get good grades.

I remember playing Pinochle with my family. I remember my dad making comments like Earth to Rick" because I was slow at deciding what card to play. But I couldn't help it when my mind was thinking about other things. I actually began wondering if there was something seriously wrong with me. I couldn't learn as easily and pick up things as quickly as some people. It was very frustrating for me. "What's wrong with me?" I kept asking myself. Keep in mind that I already had low self-esteem and very little confidence in myself.

Every time I studied, I thought I knew the material pretty well and was prepared for the test. I would flunk the test or get a D- on it. It completely devastated me. I thought I either studied the wrong material or I didn't know how to study for a test. I started asking myself, why it was so hard for me to pass a test. Was this because I was below normal intelligence? I didn't think so, but I didn't know why I had a hard time in school when trying to comprehend things.

Now I know it was because of anxiety. I wonder how many people out there right now have this problem. Some who are reading this book might be facing the same learning difficulties. Relax if you are. There is HELP TO STOP THE ANXIETY, which will slow down the CPS and, in effect, help your learning and concentration. You might be asking yourself, why some people have this problem, but many don't. A lot of it has to do with thought patterns and thinking negative thoughts. Your childhood, and how you were brought up, can and will affect your thinking. If you find yourself having this problem, talk to people, parents, and professionals. It may even be a clinical problem, which can only be treated by medication.

CHAPTER 3
Remedies for Anxiety

Here are some suggestions to stop anxiety:

- If you are fearful or anxious, stand in front of a mirror and tell yourself, I am really joyful!" Act and keep acting until it becomes a part of you. Tell yourself from now on that you are going to live most of your time with a joyful attitude.

- Another method is through meditation. Without distractions, sit quietly and breathe slowly. Try to block out everything in your mind, and focus on your breathing, and count to three a couple of times. Tell yourself to relax, relax. Anxiety cannot come to a calm mind. Try this for ten minutes or so.

- Another way to stop anxiety is to eliminate negative thoughts. It is a habit that is not easy to stop, especially when you have been conditioned to this type of thinking most of your life. So how do you stop the negative thoughts from entering your mind and taking over? When the negative thoughts enter your mind, feed your brain with the opposite message. The brain cannot think of both negative and positive thoughts at the same time.

- Just say "No" or "Stop" to yourself. When the thought re-enters, say "stop" aloud. It's even better if you can do this looking in a mirror.

- Eat an apple and chew it slowly, really concentrating on the flavor of the apple.

- Along with the apple, drink a glass of water.

- Eat lettuce slowly. Focus your attention on the lettuce. If your mind strays, bring it back to what you are doing presently.

- Picture in your mind a color of choice and give it a shape.

- Close both eyes and hold both ears: try to imitate a bird or hear a chirp.

Finally, one of the best ways to heal the mind is with laughter. Watch funny movies and laugh. Laughter changes the chemicals in the brain and is also a healing inhibitor. There has been a noted case of a very sick person going into a hospital with little chance of survival. After watching nothing but funny films and cartoons and laughing for a period of time, the patient came out healed. So, laugh, even if you must force yourself. It has been proven that laughter heals people.

You may also want to try these techniques:

- Stand before mirror and make faces with laughter no less than twice a day until anxiety stops.

- When negative thoughts enter your mind sit down with yourself and discuss them verbally along with any fears you have.

- Breathe slowly at least twenty minutes a day in a comfortable position.

- Watch the flickering of a candle for twenty or thirty minutes without moving or losing concentration.

- Don't get anxious on anxiety. Tell yourself to let the monster starve.

- Write down your blessings and after sing aloud.

- Slap yourself because it discharges clogged energy in you.

These exercises were given by Dr.Talib Kafaji clinical psychologist.

These exercises will help a lot, depending on the amount of your anxiety. If you are already in a depression, you certainly should seek professional help. These are good exercises, but you still may need medicine depending on the chemical situation in your brain.

I only listed a few techniques to help you overcome anxiety. I hope you find them useful.

It is also very important that you watch what you eat. Avoid sugar and sweets as much as possible because sugar helps add to anxiety. Eat lots of fruit and drink lots of water.

CHAPTER 4

The Happening

And then it happened! One day in tenth grade, I woke up and tried to get out of bed and I almost fell. My legs were partially numb and tingly. I had a hard time walking and balancing. My older brother carried me to the couch. My urinary tract stopped for two days. I was not able to urinate. The first day, my mother took me to the doctor's office; he couldn't find anything physically wrong. The next day I had the exact same symptoms. I went back to the doctor's again. He could not find anything wrong again. He thought it might be a muscle spasm and told me to soak in the bathtub.

I stayed the same way the whole day. I barely could walk. I still had the tingling in my legs and the heels of my feet were numb. Emotionally, I was scared. I did not know what was going on. For three days in a row, I woke up the same way. I had exactly the same symptoms. I was really scared this time. Again, I went to see the doctor. That was my third day without urinating so the doctor put a catheter in me. I remember how uncomfortable of a feeling that was just being in the doctor's office made me nervous enough. This problem added to the anxiety. He also admitted me to the hospital because there was nothing else he could do. It was, at the time, one of the best hospitals around, with the best doctors who were trained in special areas.

They ran test after test, and all the tests came back negative. I saw specialist after specialist, and they still could not find anything wrong with me. I remember the doctors telling my parents that I was being paralyzed. They decided to do a spinal tap, but that too came back normal. Imagine being fifteen years old and, at one time, one of the fastest runners in school, and you have to deal with the thought that you may not walk again. What an emotional shock to the mind and body. This is what I was going through without all the facts plus my mind would make things much worse than they really were. It turned out they had made a mistake in reading my test.

After three weeks of examination nothing was found, so they decided I would be better off at home. I think they came to the conclusion it was brought upon from inside, emotionally, and decided I would be better off at home. They released me from the hospital. I went once or twice for outpatient psychological counseling. Now I realize I should have continued in counseling for a long time.

I missed three weeks of school. A good academic person would have found it almost impossible to make the work up, but how much harder would it be for me in my emotional state? At least I could walk, but there was still numbness in parts of my legs. It took about a year and a half before all the numbness and tingling went away. If I had had the proper nurturing and self confidence, it may not have manifested itself the way it did.

When I went back to school, I felt strange. This was The first time I had been out of school in a long time. I had an almost perfect attendance record all the way through school, previous to this. I knew I was flunking bookkeeping and I was barely getting by on some other classes. I was required to take a physical education class in tenth grade. But due to my problem, I had a critical excuse but I would have to make it up my senior year in order to graduate. Self-pity is the wrong course to take. Unknowingly, I had brought this problem on myself. I needed to love myself. I needed, at this point, to change my whole process of negative thinking to positive thought. I did not love myself. I did not have control over my thoughts. I needed to be kind to my inner child (myself) and I wasn't.

Kids must develop SELF ACCEPTANCE and SELF CONFIDENCE. Just like the song goes, "Without Love I am nothing, without love for yourself and others, that is.

So, what was my diagnosis? I don't think they knew for sure. It was not related to any physical problem it all came from emotion. As you know the mind and body work together.) I know the psychological term for what happened is called somatoform disorder. The somatoform disorders are a group of mental disturbance placed in a common category on the basis of their external symptoms. These disorders are characterized by physical complaints that appear to be medical in origin but that cannot be explained in terms Of a physical disease. Perhaps the results of substance abuse or of another mental disorder. In order to meet the criteria for a somatoform disorder, the physical symptoms must be serious enough to interfere with the patient's employment or relationships, and must be symptoms that are not under the Patient's voluntary control. General, somatoform disorders are characterized by disturbances in the patient's physical sensations or ability to move the limbs or walk.

This disorder can also be a condition in which the patient's senses or ability to walk or move are impaired without a recognized medical or neurological disease or cause; and in which psychological factors (such as stress or trauma) are judged to be temporarily related to onset or exacerbation. The disorder gets its name from the notion that the patient is converting a psychological conflict or problem into an inability to move specific parts of the body or to use his or her senses normally. The symptom simultaneously contains the anxiety and serves to get the patient out of the threatening situation. The physical symptoms of conversion disorder may include a loss of balance or paralysis of an arm or leg; the inability to swallow or to speak; the loss of touch or pain sensation going blind or deaf seeing double, or having hallucinations, seizures, or convulsions.

This was the first time in my life that the emotional problems manifested physically. Little did I know that this was the start of many physical ailments? The older I got, the more the physical symptoms increased.

If parents really knew how important it is to nurture and admonish their children while they're growing up ,and if they followed through with it there would be a lot less children hurting children today. Children and young adults have so much anger in them. They release their anger by shooting and killing people because they have never been made whole or emptied their garbage can emotionally.

At some point and time the pattern has to stop. The cycle of raising unhealthy children must be broken and the problem will correct itself. What we have in America today are (children, emotionally speaking) raising children. What I mean is people who are not healthy emotionally and have childhood issues that have never been resolved in their own life and some of their behaviors are passed on to their own offspring. The result is you have kids growing up with anger, not Knowing why they are angry, and not knowing whom it is they are angry at.

My senior year was much improved. First, I became involved in drama and was in a play called *The Man Who Came to Dinner*. I had a minor role. I played the butler and had about ten speaking lines, but it really gave me some confidence. I remember going to practice at night during the week. It kept me occupied and I felt like one of the crowd. For the first time in many years, I felt like a normal student and that I wasn't different. What a morale booster.

A lot of the students would drive to and from rehearsal, but I would either walk or have my dad take me. This really bothered me a lot because my dad would not let me and my brothers or sister drive the car. It was normal for a teenager to use his parent's car to go places I really wanted and needed to drive. His dad died when he was eight or nine years old, so he didn't have someone to talk to growing up. His parents both came from Poland. You might say they were from the old school, so my dad grew up with a lot of" garbage feelings "and no one there to help correct his thought patterns. Can you imagine your dad dying at eight or nine years old and not getting psychological or emotional help? What an effect it must have had on him all his life. What a shock to a little kid. He didn't have a dad anymore, and was without help in society. Needless to say, he must have carried with him a lot of emotional emptiness and loneliness all his life. Back in the 1920s, you didn't get the help and support groups, we have now. He, along with many other people grew up without getting feelings and issues resolved or fixed. A lot of emotional needs were not met.

As I said, I became involved in drama and I began working part time at night and on weekends. I began to get some self-esteem back and gain some confidence. The year continued to go by fast. For the first time in six years, I felt like I was one of the crowd. Amazing what a mind in control can do. As May drew closer, so did graduation. With my good grades, my involvement in school activities, and my part-time job, I felt good. If only the rest of my years could have gone like my senior year.

Well, graduation quickly came and went. The cap and gown came off. Then on graduation night, as I sat in a restaurant with my mom, the scary feelings came back. The summer continued, I started to work full time. I purchased my very first car and the good feelings started up again and continued. I had made some accomplishments, I had self-esteem, I was working full time at a decent paying job, and I had my own car.

It went well for a year and a half and then I met the girl with whom I would fall in love and eventually marry. I needed to learn how to let things roll off of my back like a duck, but it was hard for me to do. It was hard because I had an inordinate love for people and a need to be loved. In the years to come, I would again go through some of the worse times of my life.

There I was, nineteen years old and falling in love and then I got a draft notice. This was during the Viet Nam War. I did not want to go into the armed forces. Several of my friends were enlisting, and at that time, it seemed to be the thing to do. You either went to college or enlisted in the armed forces. I'll never forget that bus ride from Fort. Wayne, MI to Fort.. Knox, KY. All I could do was stare out the window, thinking about my girlfriend and how I would miss her ,and keeping her picture close to my heart. Physically, I was on the bus, but my heart was with her..

This, by far, would be the worst shock to my system. Can you imagine what I was going through? My life was completely out of my control. I couldn't stand the fact that I couldn't do what I wanted to do. When we stopped for lunch on the bus ride to Fort Knox I completely lost my appetite. (I completely lose my appetite when I am under anxiety. My system seems to shut down and I can go for a long time without eating.) My anxiety was really high and I cried fervently and prayed to God that if he got me home I would be obedient. I prayed day and night asking God to get me home. I knew that God was more powerful than any nation, Army, or person .That He definitely was in control no matter how impossible the situation seemed. After the third week of basic training, I developed a hernia. They gave me the option of having it rectified and staying in the Army or getting a medical discharge.

I came back home and went back to my normal life. I continued dating the same girl who would become my wife in 1973. Before we got married, I kept my promise to God. I got involved with bible studies; it changed my life and I became a Christian. I got married and I bought a mobile home. During this time, I tried to go to college part-time, but I still couldn't focus. I continued on with my way of life. I had a hard time figuring things out because of the abnormal brain waves, which caused me anxiety. It was a big change, being married. I had more responsibility and I had left my comfort zone. But in a lot of ways, it was good for me. For one of the first time in my life, I felt like I was in control. I had to be responsible for a wife, a place to live, and a job. I thought I was doing pretty well for myself.

Two years after we were married, my wife became pregnant and the fear started up again. This time it was about having a child. It was the same fear in the beginning of my story. My mind kept obsessing about having a baby. I didn't know, at that time, if I had the tools to be a parent. It was scary for me to think about having a child. It's a tremendous responsibility to bring up a child so that when he or she grows up, he or she will be an emotionally healthy and moral person, making right decisions.

Once again, I had to leave my comfort zone. I didn't know why it was so hard for me to accept changes. I just knew that from the time I was young, I had that problem.

I had a son, who I became very close to later in life Together we've built a great relationship. It's a relationship that I am very proud of..Two years after my son was born, we had a daughter, who at that time was my joy. I always wanted her to be daddy's little girl. My children are my pride and joy.

As time moved on, my thoughts became harder and harder to control and little things started bothering me more. The anxiety and obsessive thoughts bothered me so much that it soon started affecting me physically again. I became nauseated at times. As time progressed, my stomach problems led to spastic colitis. (That is when your bowel gets irritated and it can make you sick.) So I battled with that for a year. I can remember how bad it used to make me feel. I never felt like doing anything. I guess a good description of it would be much like having the flu. I looked perfectly healthy, but I felt so bad. There was a constant churning in my stomach. So many times, I felt like I would vomit but never did. It took me a few years to realize that my physical problems were caused by emotional stress. I soon realized that negative thoughts plus negative feelings equaled physical symptoms; I believe that many people today would have a lot less stress and problems if they would get rid of anger, envy, and bitterness. Those things create poison in your body. It's rottenness to the bones. If people would eliminate these feelings, that could eliminate a lot of medical problems.

CHAPTER 5

My Pride and Joy

W e only lived two blocks away from the school. Which was nice so that the kids could walk instead of having to take a bus or get a ride. The first day my son went to school he looked so scared? This would be his first time away from his mom and dad. In fact, as I write this, I can recall my first experience walking to school for the first time I wanted my mom to go to school with me. As my son left for school, I could relate to exactly how he was feeling. I wished I could have gone with him, but I couldn't, so I just waved goodbye to my little guy as the bus went down the street. I'm sure almost all parents go through those emotions.

When my son was old enough to play baseball, I went with him to every practice and every game. I helped him the best I could. Maybe I caused too much pressure and made him nervous, but I was just trying to give my boy what I never got from my dad. I was reliving my life through him. I can remember my daughter in the sixth grade working in the office at the school .One day she called from the office doing some work there. That was something I will never forget because she had that responsibility and made me feel proud of her.

It was so neat to see both of our children go to all of the same schools we went to. Anyway, back to reality. Life went on and the kids got older. I enjoyed my kids as they were growing up. I especially liked it when they started band in the seventh grade. They were in band all the way to graduation.

CHAPTER 6

Depression

U p until this time I did not have a major depression episode. However I did know that at times there were mood swings. This seemed to cycle. I did not know until years later I would be diagnosed being bi-polar which I will explain later. As I approached forty, I received a promotion at the grocery store, managing the dairy department. I didn't have much help and I would get mad because there was too much to do. I found out quickly that if you don't speak up and stand up for yourself some companies take advantage of you.

I have always been one that does not like conflict. That has been a big part of my problem and not standing up for myself and that creates anger.. Once, while in the cooler, I got so mad that I felt something in my head actually move. I actually felt a click. I asked the doctor about it later. He said some people do experience a type of click in the head when a depression episode begins. What I was about to go through, no person should have to experience, it was like living in a deep black hole. I could not figure out what was wrong. My problem was both physical and emotional. My whole body broke down. I was sick, nauseated, so tired, and could not concentrate at all. I lost all happy feelings. I could not enjoy anything at all. I completely lost my appetite. I had no desire to go anywhere or do anything. I did not want to get up in the morning. All I wanted to do was go to bed, but I could not sleep because my mind was jumping around from thought to thought. It was like I had brain-lock. I could not think about anything else except what happened.

I ended up going to the University of Michigan outpatient clinic once a month for about eighteen months. I was diagnosed with massive depressive syndrome. Depression, I think is one of the worse illnesses in the world. Most people, unless they have been through it themselves, cannot relate to what a person goes through when he or she is in a state of depression. What is really aggravating is the fact that you look healthy and normal to other people, but you feel so terrible. People don't understand.. A person can read all the books they want, talk to people who have been in the situation, or have all the medical degrees there are, but the conclusion is nobody knows what it is like living in a depression unless they have experienced it. In many cases laughter will help. In chronic cases laughter may not help depending how severe the episode is. A lot of prescriptions just sedate you and keep you functional.. Since depression is caused by a chemical change in the brain, the proper medicine will help you, but it takes time for the brain to get back into normal function. There are some people that never will overcome severe depression.. For those people life can be a constant battle to survive.

You get tired of living this way real quick. Fears become exaggerated. Negative thoughts can magnify themselves immensely. You are really tired all the time . I did not have the slightest thought of suicide. Now I see why people take their lives. I do not advocate or condone suicide, but I can understand why some people do it, especially if they're without God because without Him there often is no hope.

Depression is like falling into an abyss. You see yourself tumbling down into it and you stretch out your hands to other people. They reach out their hand to grasp yours but they are inches apart and cannot quite connect with you. And yet you can see each other. There you are, hopeless and alone. All they can do is watch. You can see them eye-to-eye, but they cannot help. All you want to do is cry, and not be left alone. I think loneliness is the worst feeling in the world. You feel so lonely and no one can help. You try to laugh at things, but you must force yourself. It does not work for long. It may work for a few minutes, but then those terrible feelings of loneliness and worthlessness come back. From what I have discovered, the thoughts bring on the feelings. Some medicines work for some people and not for others. Behavioral modification could have great benefits for some people, but for others it could have little effect.

After I left U.F.M. clinic I found my own psychiatrist. I also started getting psychological training from Dr. Talib, who was a clinical psychologist. He was the one I mentioned earlier who gave me some tools to help overcome anxiety. He helped me with a lot of my negative thoughts. In fact, he was the one who encouraged me to write a book on anxiety from a patient's perspective. Because when I started checking around for material to read, I couldn't find much on the subject from a personal view. I decided to write my own book t o help millons of people out there suffering. I continued to the best of my ability to work. About one year later the depression subsided and I started living again instead

Of just getting up and going through the motions. The emotional feelings were gone and for the most part my life was back to normal. People need to appreciate when you can go through daily live without fears and emotional problems.

After having another incident at work, which affected me so badly and caused

so much anxiety and anger because I was treated unfairly and not standing up for myself I had to take the whole summer off. Emotionally I could not work.. There I was off work, sitting on the park bench. As I wrote this, I'm recalled how much I missed my dad while I was growing up. If only he had come to some of my baseball games. As I would go up to the plate, I always looked for my dad, especially after I made a good play in the infield, where I usually played third base or shortstop.

How I missed you dad. Why didn't you come to my baseball games? Now I hurt because "little Ricky" missed you so much. I wanted you to be so proud of me but you were not there. I looked around and saw a lot of other fathers there, but you were not one of them. I asked you several times to come to some of my games, but you did not know how important it was to me. I'll never see you or touch you again. If only you had been there to support me. I was proud of myself because I was a good player and I couldn't share that with you. That meant so much to me and the sad part is you will never know because I never told you. Every time I read this, it brings tears to my eyes and I feel a loneliness that only you could have filled. However he did the best he could without a father.

I found I could do my best writing and thinking outside in the woods where there is peace and serenity.

No one knows how his or her life is going to turn out. That is why we need to make the most of every day and try to do something for humanity at every opportunity we get. Just live from day to day and enjoy life the best way you can. Life is not good or bad. Life is what we make of it. It is the mind's reaction to what happens in life.

Sometimes I wish I could have had a brain operation to take all fear and anxieties away. I think the day will come when they can remove part of the brain that causes depression and anxieties. I think most of it comes from the prefrontal cortex. The part of the brain from where emotion comes. My neurotransmitters were not functioning the way they should have. Sometimes I have brain-lock where I cannot stop thinking about a particular thing no matter what I try.. I must feed my brain with all the positive attributes I have in my life, such as family and church. I use to sing in a barbershop chorus. We would sing at senior citizen's homes. A lot of them were bed ridden and our voices would be the last voice that some hear as they are about to pass from this life. There is no greater feeling you can get out of life when you know that you have touched someone so deeply on his or her deathbed. Singing to someone can have such an effect, not just on his or her life but yours also. Expressing this kind of love to people is one of those things that matters the most in this world. It is amazing what singing can do for a person. It has been proven that a person who likes to sing and sings a lot can add a few years to his or her life. It is one of those innate qualities that human beings are made of. I believe singing can help induce some of the chemicals in the brain that can help lead to longevity. Because mind and body work together, positive affirmations in the brain can help fight off physical ailments that might occur if it were not for singing.

CHAPTER 7

Unconditional Love

I really like animals, especially dogs. I tried my own business of pet sitting several times, but it did not work out. I know how animals can help people emotionally. Dogs and cats give unconditional love. It has been proven that when seniors have animals around them to love and comfort them, they are happier and more content, and some people could live longer than those without pets. The saying is true and speaks for itself that Dog is a man's best friend. I love animals; they are pretty neat and have a lot of the feelings that people have. They also have the senses that we have and I think they have some that people don't have. When my dog was younger, he would take off down the street when he saw a squirrel. He was so fast that when the door was opened you couldn't stop him.

My dad really liked my dog. Whenever I went to visit my father, sometimes I brought my dog. My dad would always feed him and pet him. Sometimes my dad would buy something special for my dog and cook it just for him. My dog really liked my dad too. They each had unconditional love for each other. My dog filled an emotional need my dad did not have.

I remember when my dad died, the very next day my sister and I were at our childhood home, where my dad lived. Somehow, my dog had gotten out of our house. Just as my sister and I were approaching the porch to go inside, my dog was there already.

It seemed to me that my dog knew something was wrong. It was almost as if he came to the house just to see my dad. I think dogs have that extra sense of perception. I don't think it was by serendipity that my dog got there the exact same time that my sister and I did. We lived over a half mile away. I think he sensed that his other companion in life was not to be found there anymore.

My dog is getting old now, but just like people, he still wants to be loved and wants affection. Whatever room you are in, he more than likely will be there too because he loves to be with people. It doesn't seem right, but some people can get along better with dogs than they can with people. At the time of writing, my dog has been dead six years. I still think about him often, like a lot of people do when their pet dies.

CHAPTER 8

Depression

M ajor depression order is the leading cause of disability in the U.S. for people between the ages of 15-44 years.
It affects approximately 14.8 million American adults, or about 6.7% of the U.S. population age 18 and older in a given year. Although anyone can get depression, everyone does not have the same risk or experience it the same way.

Here are some signs to look for:

1. Feel sad or empty. Others have notice down mood.
2. Little interest in doing things you use to enjoy.
3. Weight loss without dieting or gained weight.
4. Having trouble sleeping or want to sleep more than usual.
5. Feeling agitated or sluggish.
6. No energy or fatigued all the time.
7. A feeling of worthlessness and guilty.
8. Problem concentrating or thinking. Having trouble making decisions.
9. Think about dying, suicide, or attempting suicide.

If you are feeling suicidal please contact the National Suicide Preservation Lifeline at 1-800-273-TALK (8255) or
Contact a health care professional immediately.

I feel sorry for all the soldiers who are right now in combat and those who come home from war. Some of them will never be the same because of what they went through. Imagine the effect it must have on those who have seen their friends and comrades get wounded or killed .Some come back home and have post traumatic stress. The chemicals in the brain could change and they may think irrational thoughts under very emotional situations, If they are not treated properly or watched it could lead to suicidal thoughts. There have been many famous people who suffered from depression and / or anxiety

You are not any less of a person because you have this illness. Most people cannot help it .They have no control over their brain functions and serotonin levels. Some people can cause depression and anxiety by themselves because of circumstances they get themselves into.

One of the most famous people that suffered from depression was Abe Lincoln! Who would have thought that he would have had this problem? A lot of people feel he was one of the best presidents the United States ever had.

I heard it stated that in the U.S., somebody commits suicide every thirty minutes. Most of these people were rational thinking people at one time. Just stop and think about it. That's forty eight people that kill themselves in a twenty four hour period. That is tragic. For the person taking his or her own life, we wonder why. What on earth could be that tough to face that you would want to die? You might even say to yourself, "I have felt just as bad as he or she did but it never occurred to me to take my life."No matter how much debt I am in, or how tragic the situation I must face, or even losing my house. The thought of taking my life never entered my mind. The reason you don't have those thoughts are because your brain cells and neurotransmitters and your serotonin level are working and producing the way they should.

**An article in the *Detroit News* from July 18, 2003 5A)
"Study links gene to depression, "stated why some people
are more vulnerable to the illness after traumatic events**

"In the scientific study, researchers analyzed the type of 5-HTT gene carried by 847 adults in New Zealand who were part of a long-term health study. There are two forms of the 5HTT gene, the long form and the short. An individual can inherit two copies of the long form, two of the short, or one of each. The researchers focused on subjects in the study who had traumatic life events over a five-year period. These events could include such things as a death in the family, a marriage break up or the loss of a job. Patients with at least a copy of the short form of 5HTT were more at risk for depressions the study found, suggesting that this form of the gene caused a heightened sensitivity to emotional stress. Patients with only the long 5HTT gene were more resistant to depression after serious emotional events and tolerated stress better. Depression was diagnosed in about 33% of the study subjects who had at least one short 5HTT gene copy and who had experienced 4 traumatic events over a 5-year period. Among those with two copies of the long form of 5HTT only 17% were diagnosed with depression after 4 traumatic events.

The conclusion they reached was the tests showed that those with even one copy of the short 5 HTT gene were almost three times more likely to think about or attempt suicide than those with only the long 5HTT. This verifies what I have been saying all along about depression being caused by a chemical or lack of chemicals, in the brain. A person has no control over this. This same article also said:

The World Health Organization has identified depression as the fourth leading cause of disease burden, which is defined as the number of year's patients must live with a disability. It is estimated that about 121,000,000 people worldwide suffer from depression. The disorder is now being diagnosed more frequently and the WHO estimates that depression will become the first cause of disease burden worldwide by 2020. Although drugs successfully treat depression in millions of people, the precise causes and controls for the disorder remain elusive. Patients often must go through a trial-and-error period before the best treatment is identified.

In another article from the *Detroit News* from April 30, 2004, the headline read: Woman, 85, who killed kids blames depression.

And yet another article from the *Detroit News* from January 18, 2004, had the headline "Fears grow over number of police suicides, "One expert said more officers kill themselves than die in the line of duty.

Robert Douglas, executive director of the National P.O.L.C.E. Suicide Foundation in Pasadena Maryland estimates that 450 U.S. law enforcement workers killed themselves in 2003 compared with 148 who died in the line of duty.

Those officers were at one time regular, rational thinking people. At one time, they would never have thought of taking their own lives. What changed in these police officers? The environment that they faced day after day could have become too real and started a negative thought process cycle. The possibility of getting killed daily, the arguments they had to stop each day, all the violence and negative influx of one bad experience after another over time, could have built up. This would affect anybody and create fears in the mind, which Could have led to a chemical change in the brain, and could have caused someone to become Manic-depressive and start thinking suicidal thoughts for the first time in their lives.

Another article, by Lindsey Tanne in the Associated Press September 2009, Depression Can Strike Children as Young as Three,'

Chicago-Depression in children as young as 3 years old is real and not just a passing Grumpy mood, according to provocative new research. The study is billed as the first to show major depression can be chronic even in very young children, contrary to the stereotype of the happy-go-lucky preschooler. Until fairly recently,", people really haven't paid much attention to depressive disorders in children under the age of 6," said lead author Dr. Joan Ruby, a psychiatrist at Washington University in St. Louis. "They didn't think it could happen...because Children under 6 were too emotionally immature to experience it: Previous research Suggested that depression affects about 2 percent of U.S. Preschoolers, or roughly 160,000 youngsters, at one time or another. But it was unclear whether depression in preschoolers could be chronic. Ruby's research team followed more than 200 preschoolers age 3 to 6, for up to two years, including 75 diagnosed with major depression. The children had up to four mental health exams during the study.

Among initially depressed children, 64 percent were still depressed or had a recurrent episode of depression six months later, and 40 percent still had problems after two years.

Overall, nearly 20 percent had persistent or recurrent depression at all four exams.

Depression was most common in children whose mothers were also depressed or had other mood disorders, and among those who had experienced a traumatic event, such as the death of a parent or physical abuse. The new study, funded by the National Institute of Mental Health and released in a August issue of *Archives of General Psychiatry* did not examine depression treatment, which is highly controversial among children so young. Some advocates say parents and doctors are too quick to give children powerful psychiatric drugs. Though sure to raise eyebrows among lay people, the notion that children so young can get depressed is increasingly accepted in psychiatry. University of Chicago psychiatrist Dr. Sharon Kirsch said the public thinks of preschoolers as carefree "They get to play. Why would they be depressed? She said. But depression involves chemistry changes in the brain that can affect even youngest with an otherwise happy life.

I read about the actor Heath Ledger who played the joker in Batman possibly committed suicide because of his depressing role he played. It could have changed his brain chemical and under normal circumstances would never have done that.

Epilogue

Several years ago, I was diagnosed as bi-polar; which could be caused of a lack of serotonin. This means you get highs and lows rather than a normal constant balance.

- Sadness

- Feelings of worthlessness

- Losing interest in things and activities you once enjoyed

- Being overcome by feelings of guilt, failure, and hopelessness

- Becoming sad and unable to concentrate, remember things, or even make simple decisions

- Experiencing physiological changes like differences in appetite or weight, energy levels, and sleep schedules

- Possibly thinking about death or suicide, in extreme cases

Bipolar patients and schizophrenics have elevated activity of an enzyme called protein Kinas C, or PKC There are about five million Americans with bi-polar disorder. The symptoms and severity of the condition vary but with the proper treatment, symptoms can be managed. Some say you must also experience high or low mood swings. I said earlier that people can be diagnosed with depression and have different symptoms. And have different results with the same medication. Just so with bi-polar disorders some will have completely different problems because there are different forms of it. Recently I have heard of people doing outrageous things and say they are bi-polar which in many cases that is true. I don't want to judge people but sometimes I think they could be making excuses for their behavior. It can become easy to blame irrational decisions and anger on bi-polar -disorders. That in turn may allow people to attach a stigma every time they hear the words bi-polar. However it does not mean that he or she will all of a sudden make inappropriate decisions. Do not think that he or she is dangerous at times; this type of thinking and stigma must stop completely. In most cases the problem is real and severe and could be very dangerous without proper help. It could lead to devastating decisions that you would not make under normal circumstances.

And Finally
You must put your mind on a leash. Control your mind and develop good patterns when you are young. This is also very critical. Never compare yourself with others. This has been my problem most of my life. Apples are not tastier than bananas; they each have their own unique flavor, just as each person has a different personality. One person is not better than the other for a long time I thought other people were better than me. This is negative and it does not help.

Never place a price tag on your humanity. Accept yourself as a loving present from God. Be kind and gentle. And non-judgmental, and especially be free of guilt to yourself.

It does not matter what job or career you have in life. Everybody is equal. A job does not define a person. The essential attributes that matter are your character, your morals, and how you treat people.

I have been on the right medicine for a few years and it makes a world of difference. In searching for a solution to this problem you must be under a Dr.s care I take Prestiq and Lexaprol. These two together really work well for me. You must be patient. It can takes months to find the right medicine and proper dosage. Always remember that everybody can respond differently to the same meds. Never be inconsistent or play with different dosage. It could have a bad effect on you.

I do not have any type of medical background or psychological studies. The information I disclosed came from my own experience and my personal studies. Most of the dialogue and experiences are my own opinion and may differ from what other people say and think. This book was in the making for eleven years, that's why there is a difference in years in some areas.

I still have fears and anxieties at times. Especially if there is a drastic change in my life. Or if I have confrontation. They can bring on anxiety attacks. I can get feeling really sick. For hours or for a few days. I found that complete distraction for a few hours can make the symptoms go away as fast as they came on. I guess that can be related to the power of the mind.

But, unless you have this problem people don't understand. Even having the right tools to know what to do still is complicated. I would like to close with this thought that prayer and the mind are the most powerful force or energy in the universe.

The End By
Richard Wyrabkiewicz
2011
E-mail polishstallion4@wowway.com